Wonderfully Made

Written and Illustrated By

Stephanie Moreland

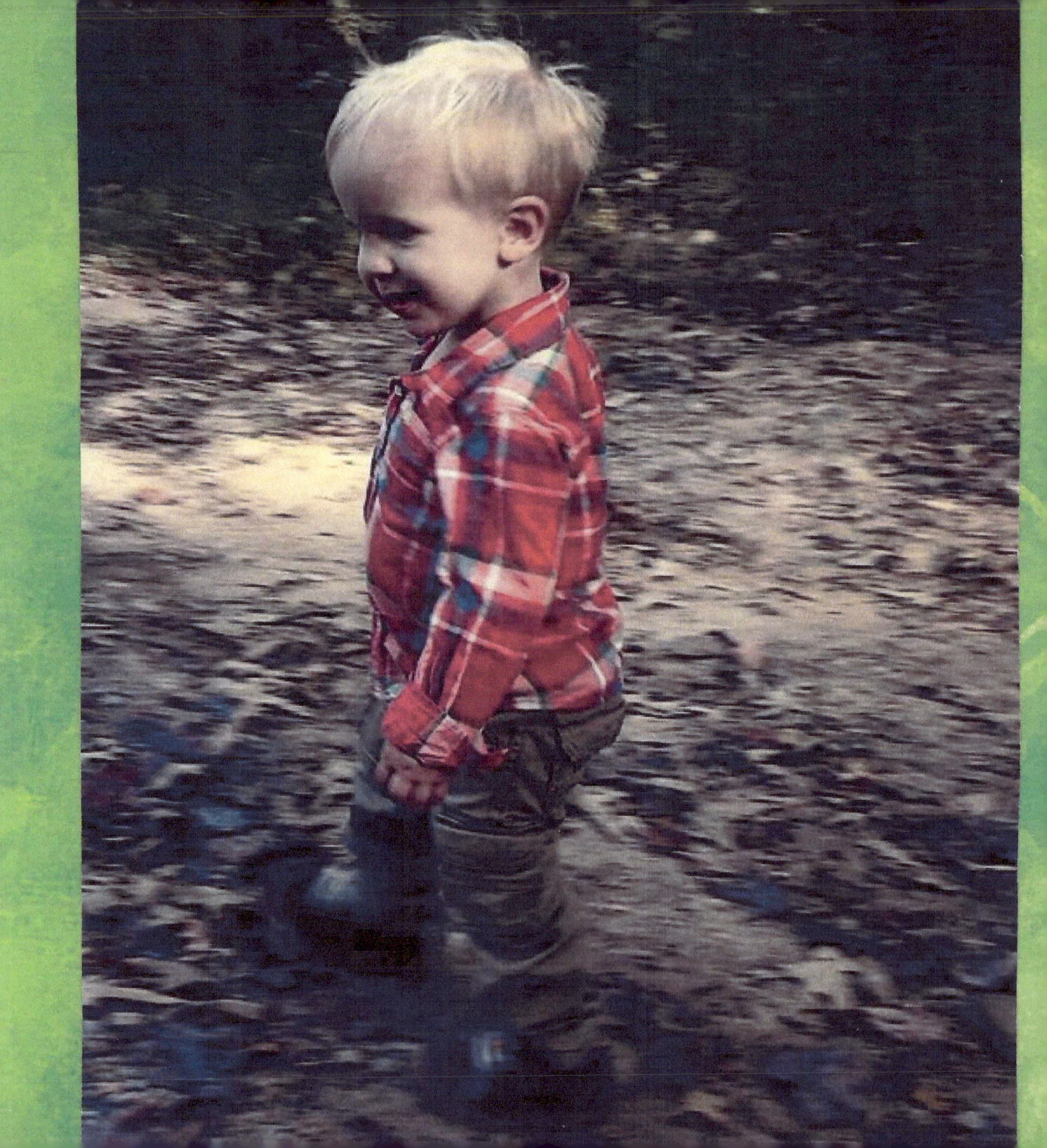

For LUKE
Your smile outshines the sun.
Your cheerful disposition and kind nature cause everyone
who meets you to instantly fall in love.

You are a blessing that God knew we needed.

We love you.

FOR ALL THE PARENTS, LIKE ME, WHO FORGOT A FEW THINGS WE LEARNED
IN HIGH SCHOOL BIOLOGY– AND NEED A LITTLE REFRESHER COURSE.

And, for all of Luke's M-CM brothers and sisters,
who have ever felt
DIFFERENt.

Once upon a time you were

VERY
SMALL.

Smaller than a seed, or grain of sand...
Smaller than a
SPECK.

You were made of just

ONE
TINY
CELL.

...And, you lived
inside my BELLY.

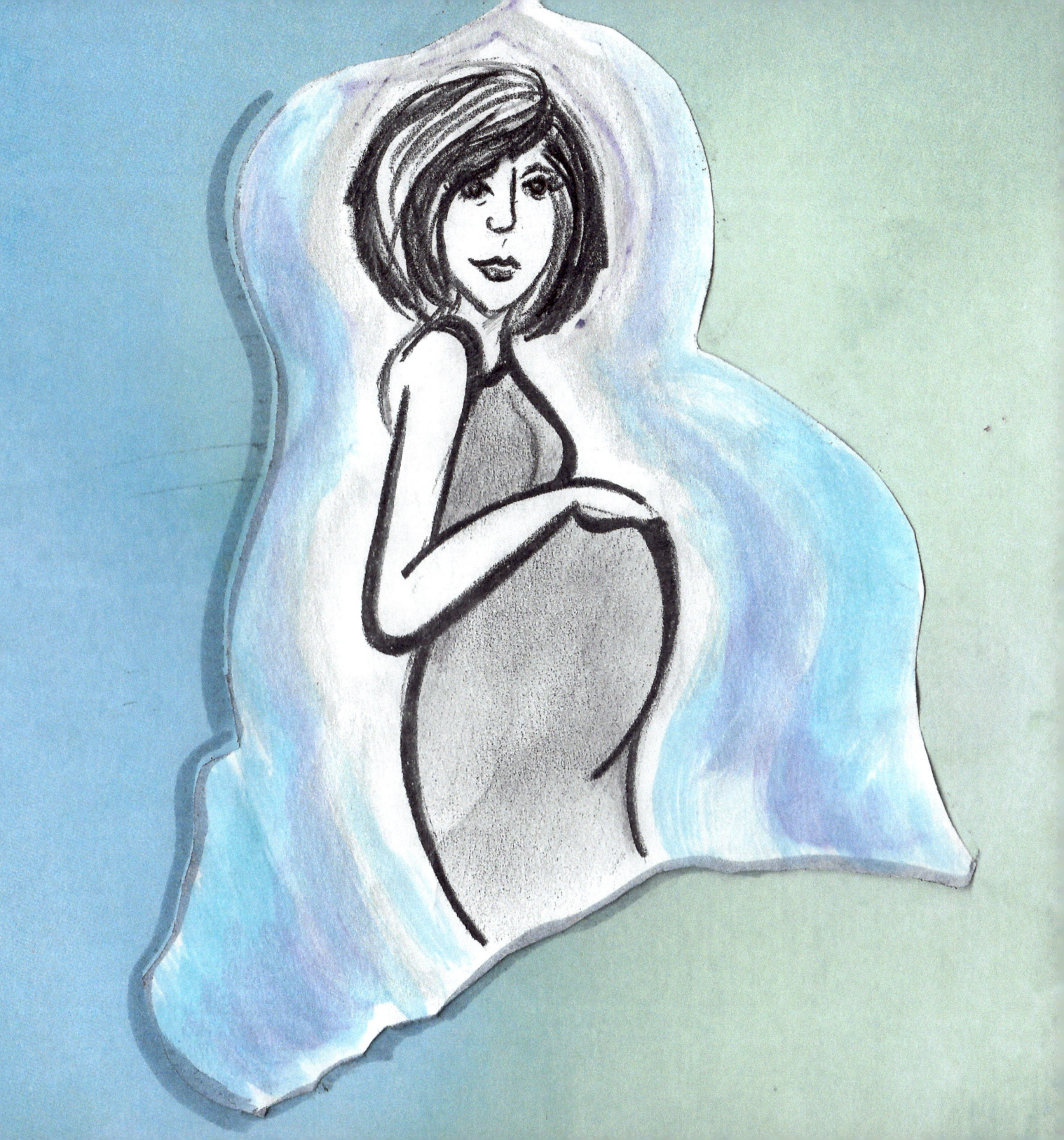

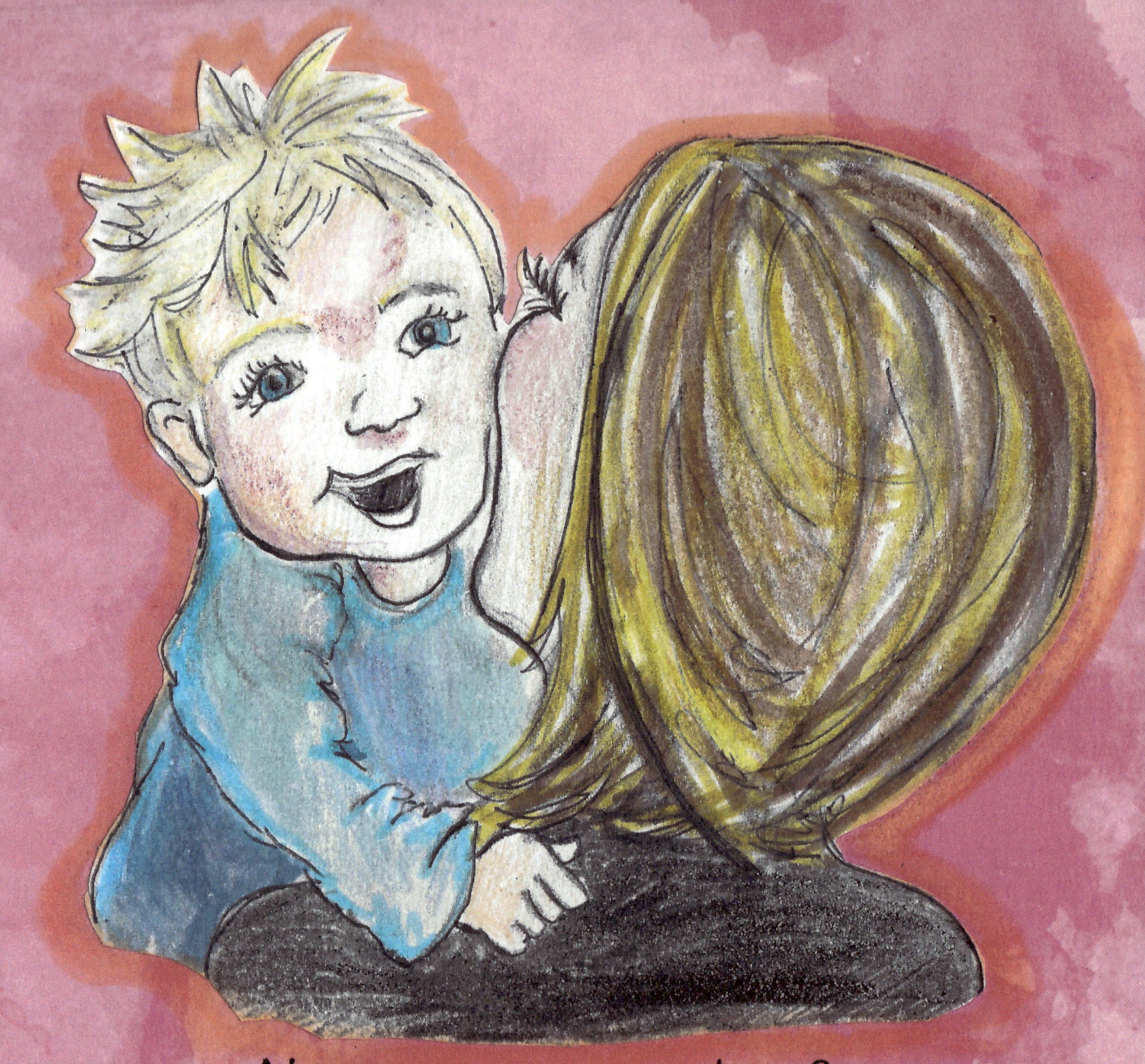

Now you are made of
one hundred thousand MILLION cells!

And guess what?!

HIDDEN INSIDE EACH AND EVERY ONE OF YOUR CELLS ARE:

(SECREt INStRUCtIoNS!!)

These instructions are called
DNA.

The DNA tells each one of your cells how to BUILD your body!

Each cell has to read the (SECREt INStRUCtIONS) to find out what to do.

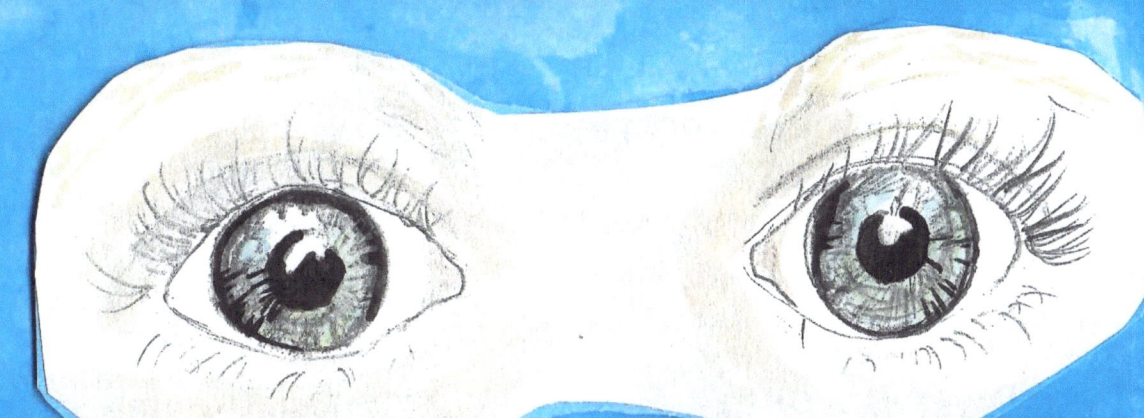

Some of the cells will tell what color to make your eyes.

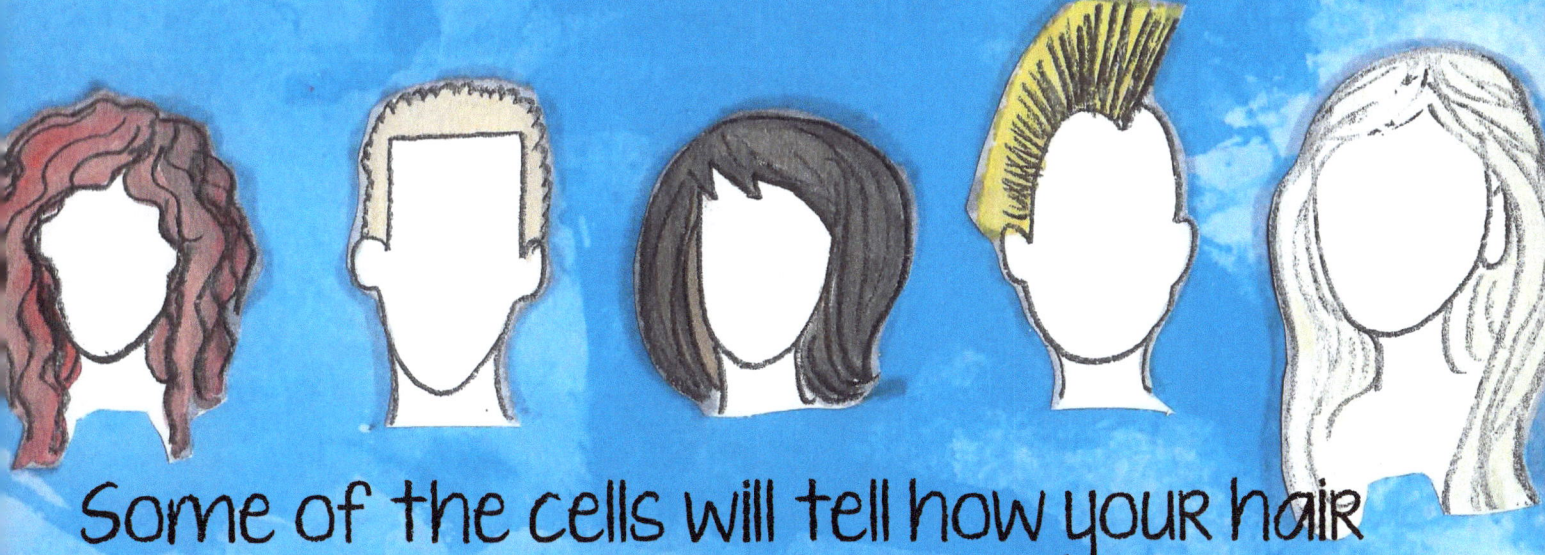

Some of the cells will tell how your hair will look.

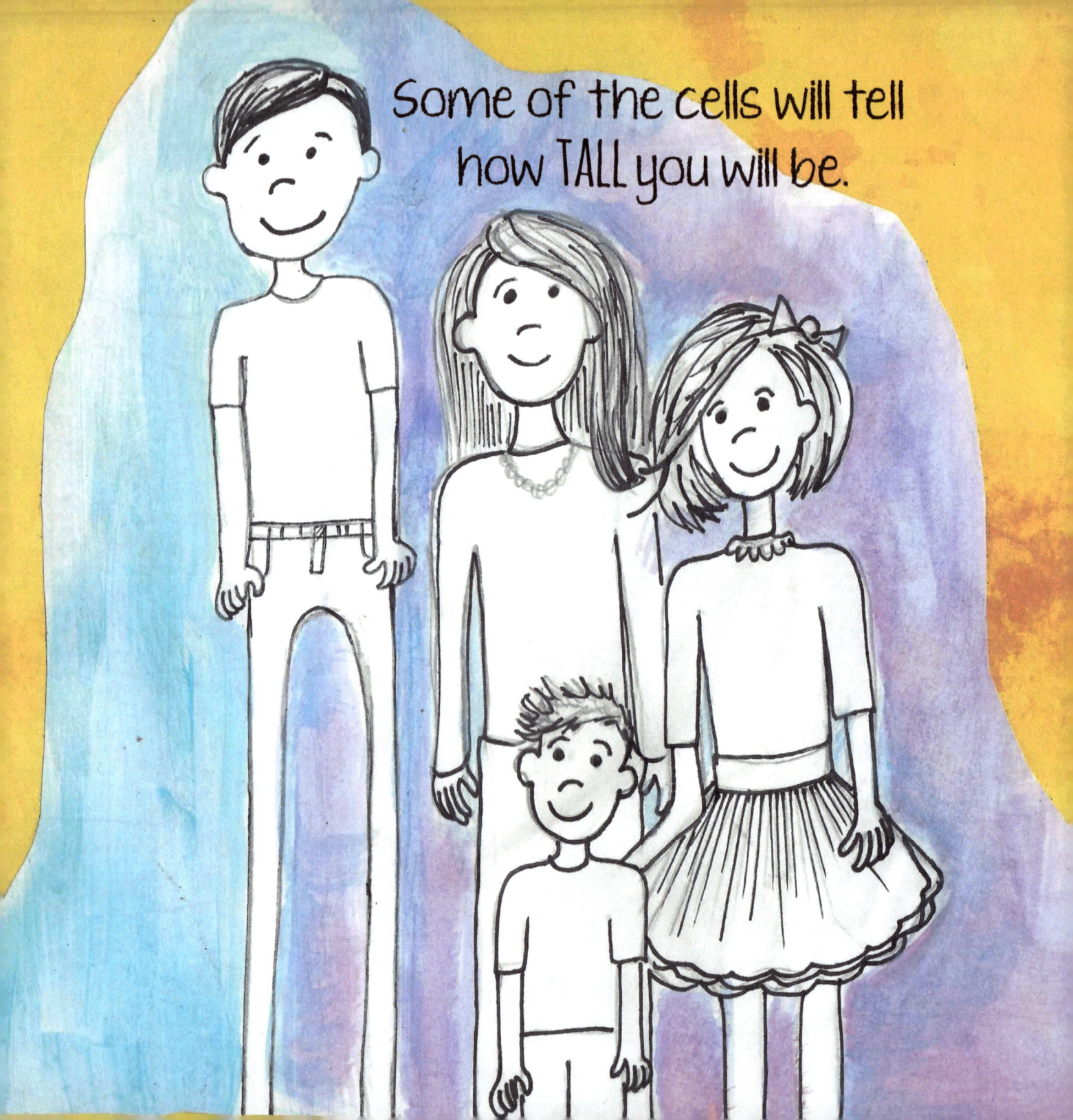

Some of the cells will tell how TALL you will be.

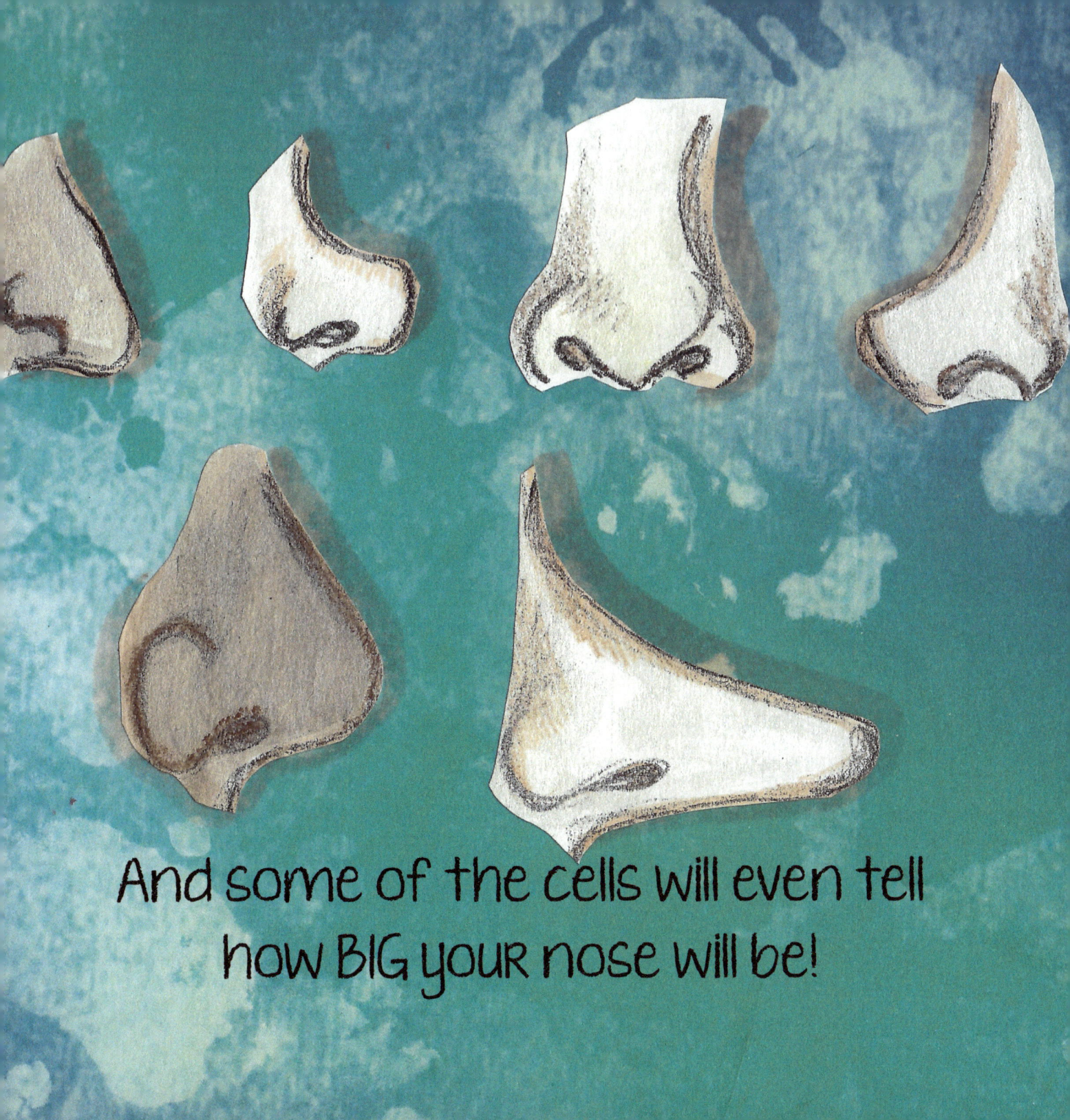

And some of the cells will even tell
how BIG your nose will be!

SHHHHH!! tOP SECREt!!

The DNA instructions....
are in a SECREt CODE!!!!
(I will give you a hint though,)
CERTAIN LETTERS ALWAYS GO TOGETHER!
A goes with T
and
C goes with G

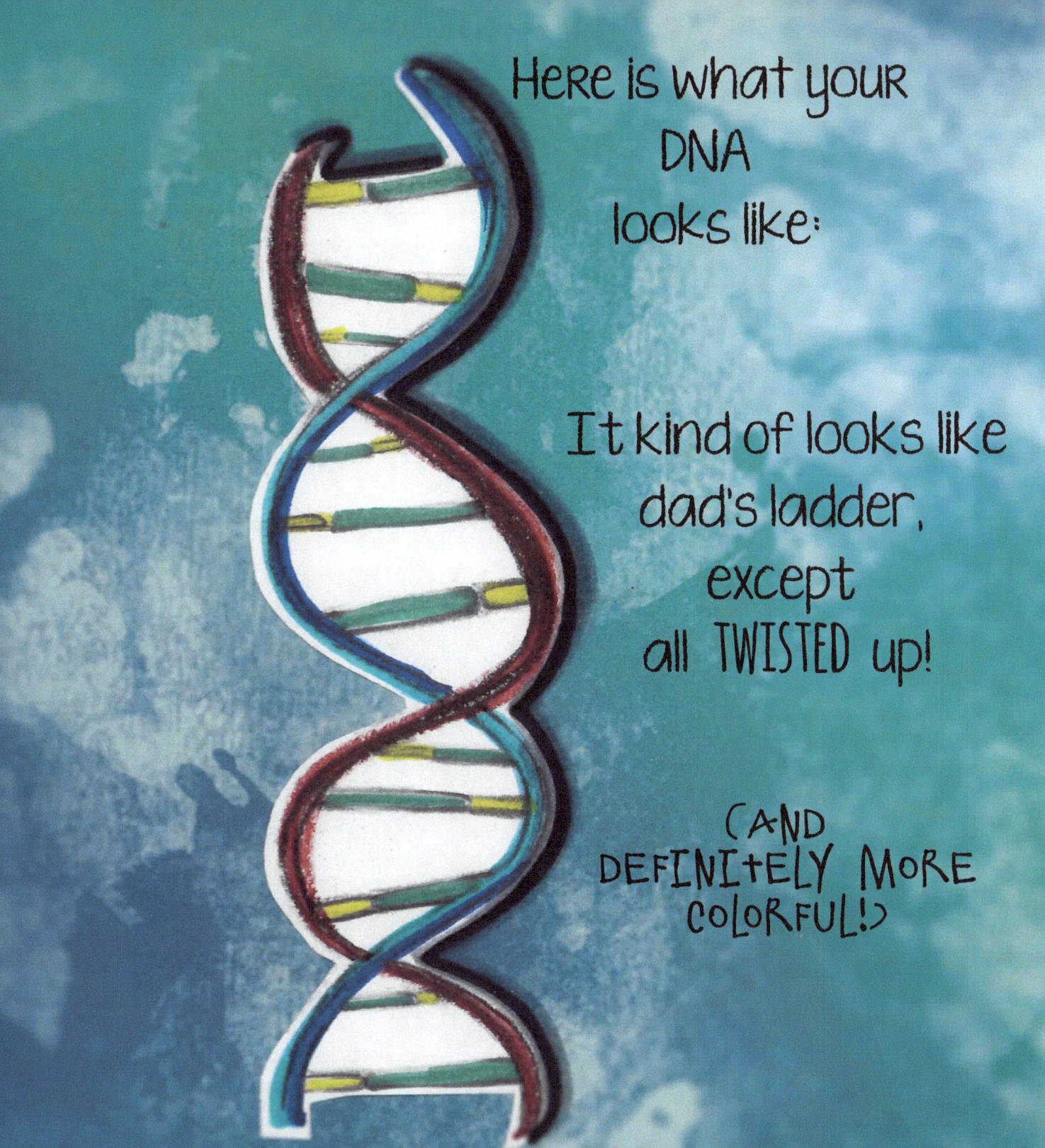

If you look at a piece
of your DNA
up close you can see
the
SECREt CODE.

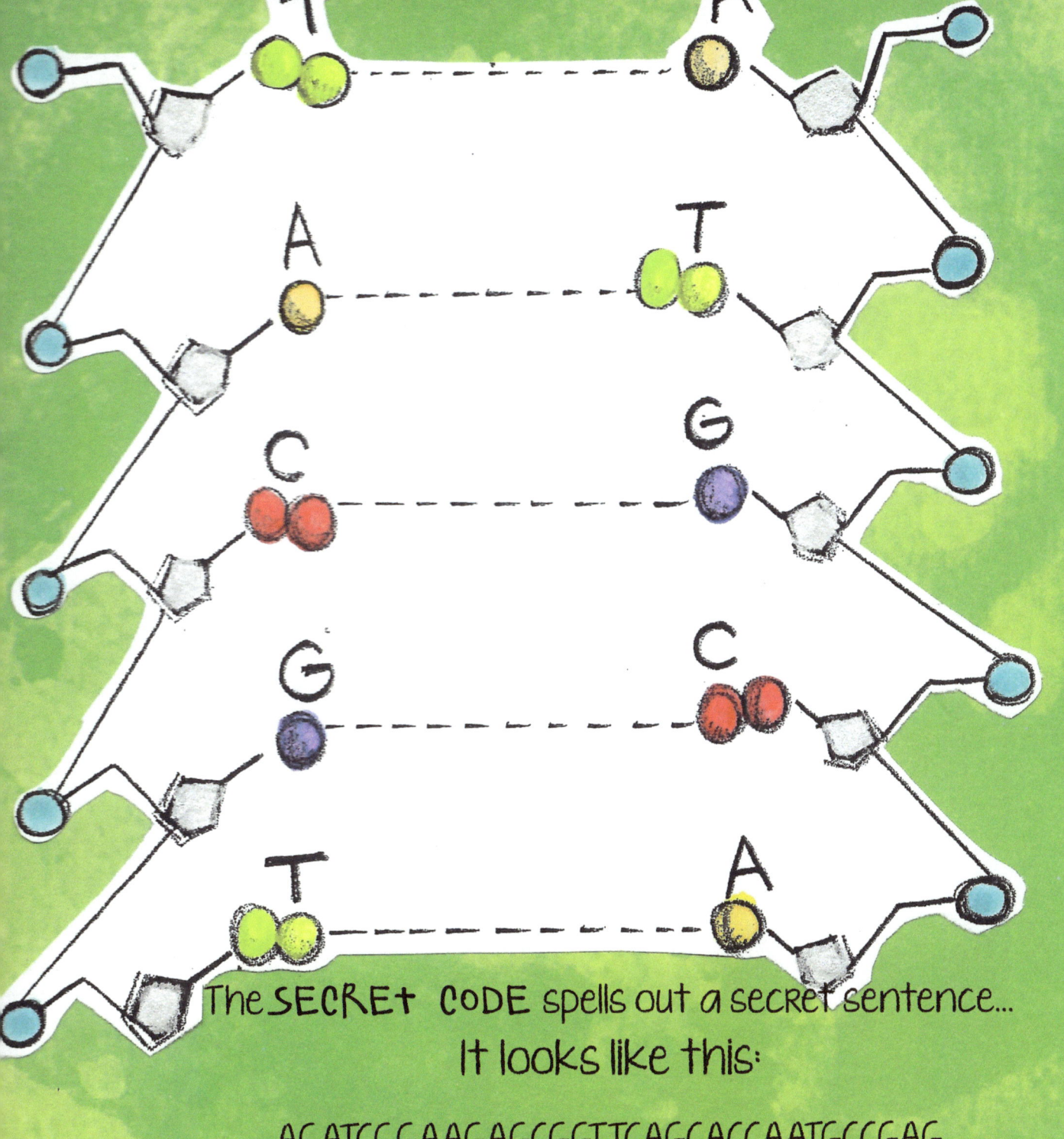

The SECREt CODE spells out a secret sentence...
It looks like this:

AGATCGGAAGAGCGGTTCAGCACCAATGCCGAG

Sometimes the
SECREt CODE
gets a little mixed up
and it
CHANGES.

tHIS IS CALLED A MUtAtION.

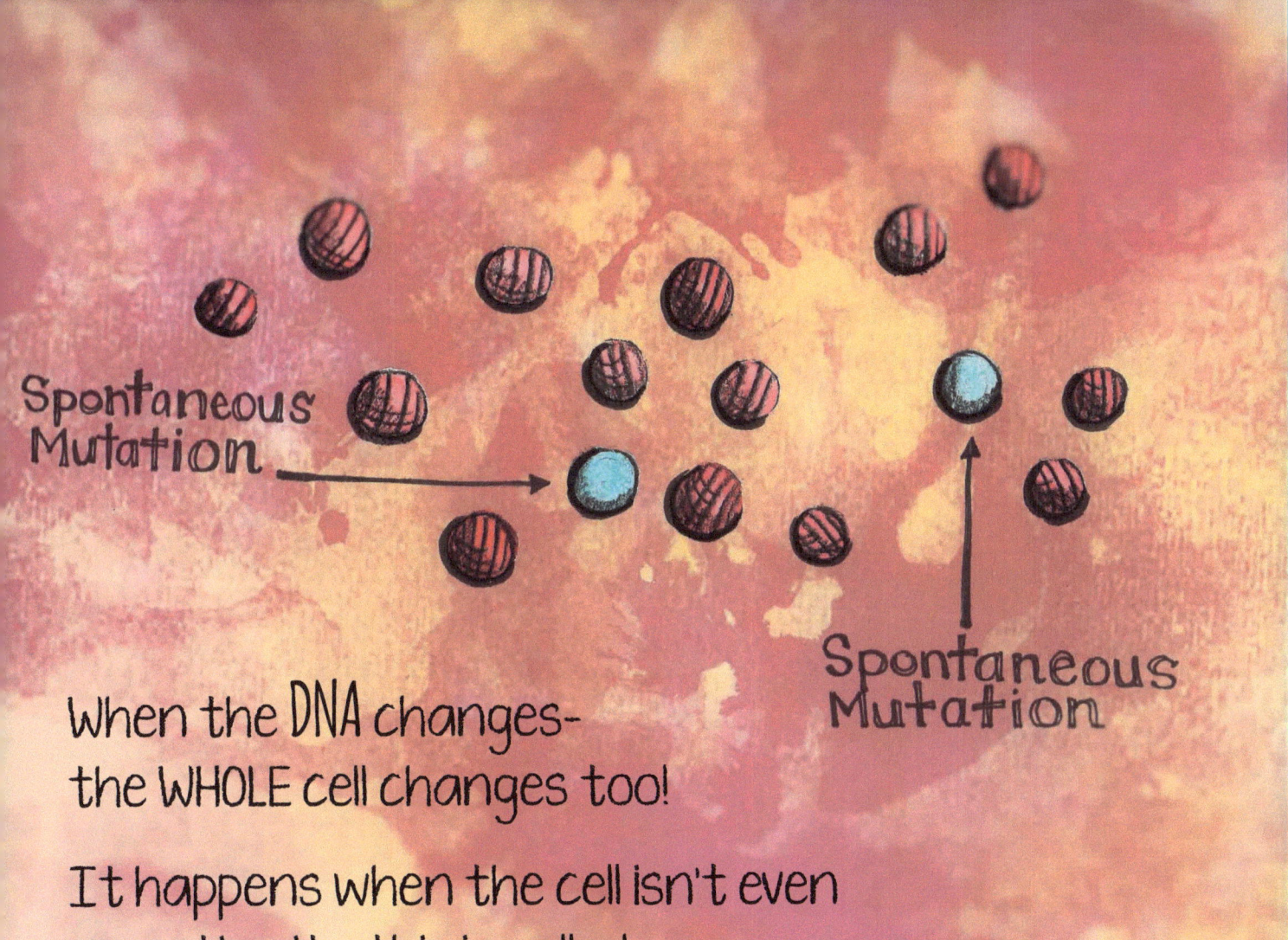

Spontaneous Mutation

Spontaneous Mutation

When the DNA changes- the WHOLE cell changes too!

It happens when the cell isn't even expecting it... this is called

SPONTANEOUS!

Read these two sentences.

The dog bit the cat.

The dog bit the car.

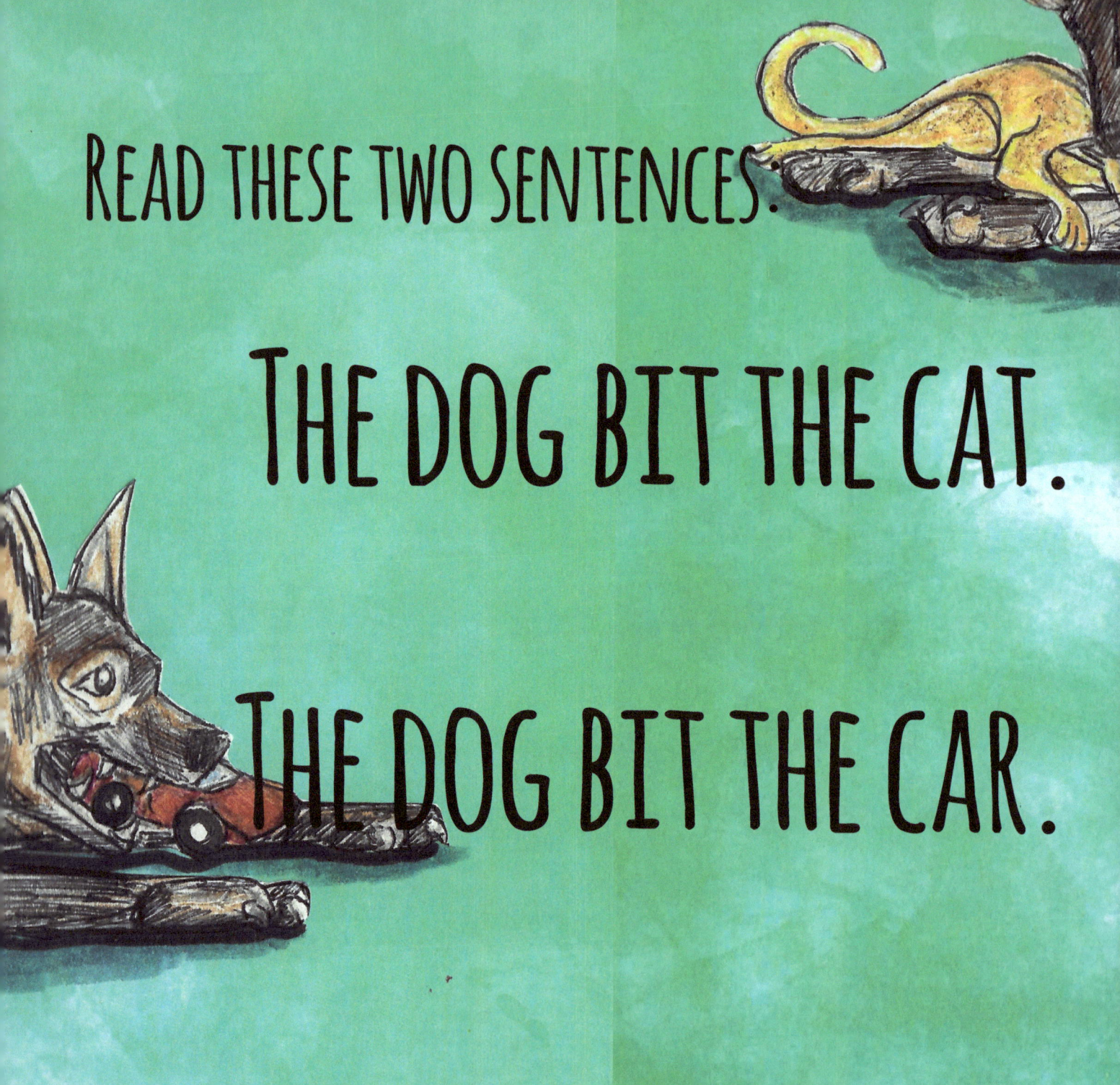

See, if you change even
just ONE letter,

it changes the meaning
of the
WHOLE sentence.

When just some of the cells
in your body are changed,
not all of them,
it is called
SOMATIC MOSAICISM.

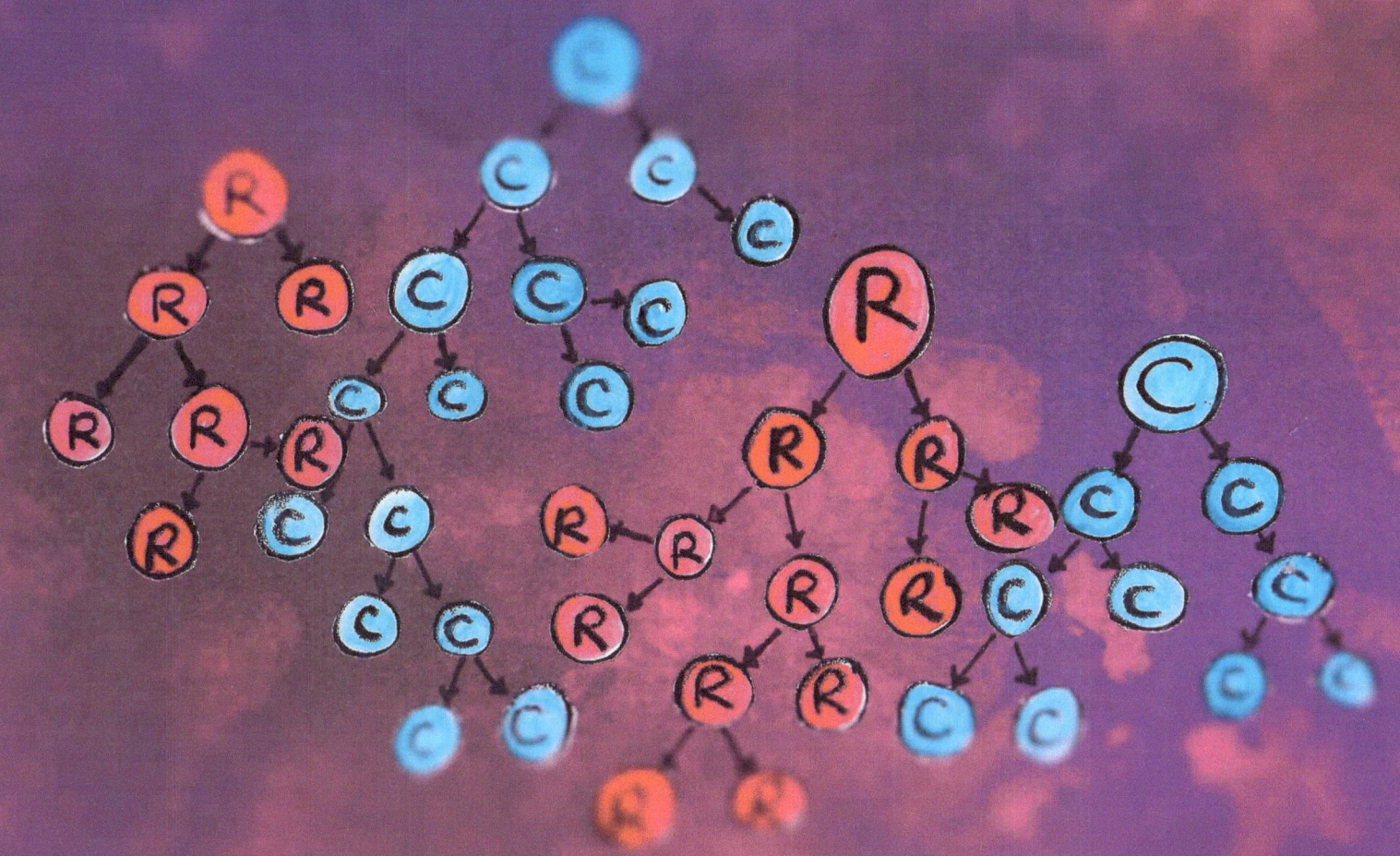

This means you have **TWO** kinds of cells now!

REGULAR AND CHANGED!

Having TWO kinds of cells sometimes means you have a "Genetic Syndrome"

such as

Macrocephaly- Capillary Malformation

(OR M-CM)

With M-CM, some of the cells are CHANGED,

(Remember: The SECREt CODE
got a little mixed up!)

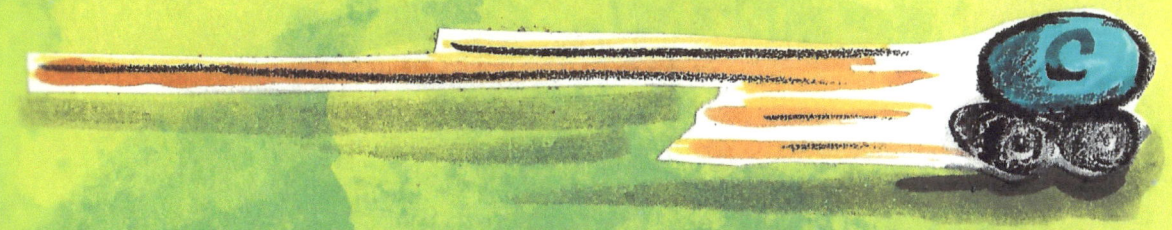

and some of the cells are regular.
And the CHANGED cells are
stronger and tougher!
And they grow and divide- and GROW and

GROW...
FASTER
than the regular cells do!

So the parts of your body that develop

from the cells that are
CHANGED

grow differently
than the parts of your body

that develop

from the cells that are
REGULAR.

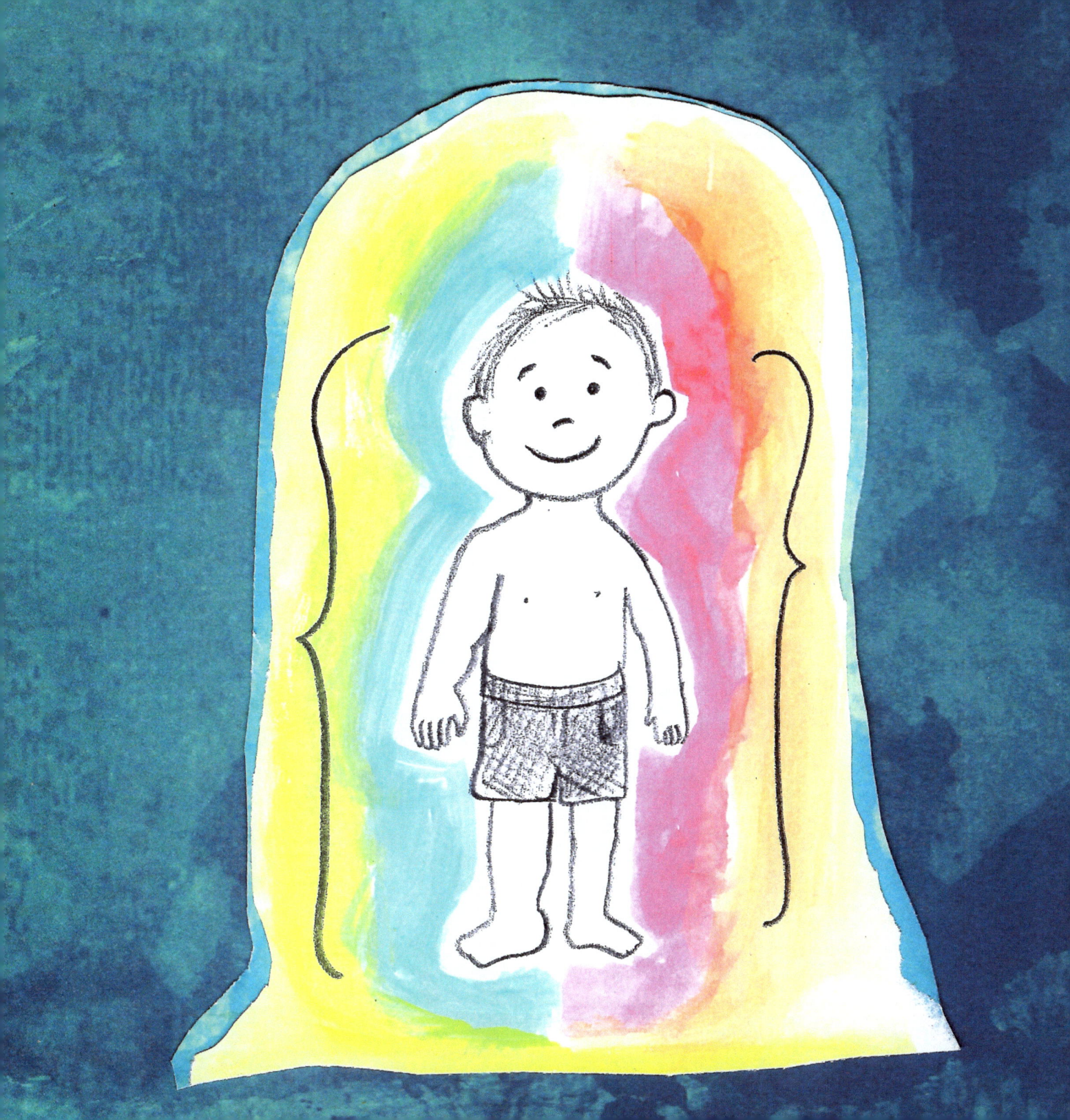

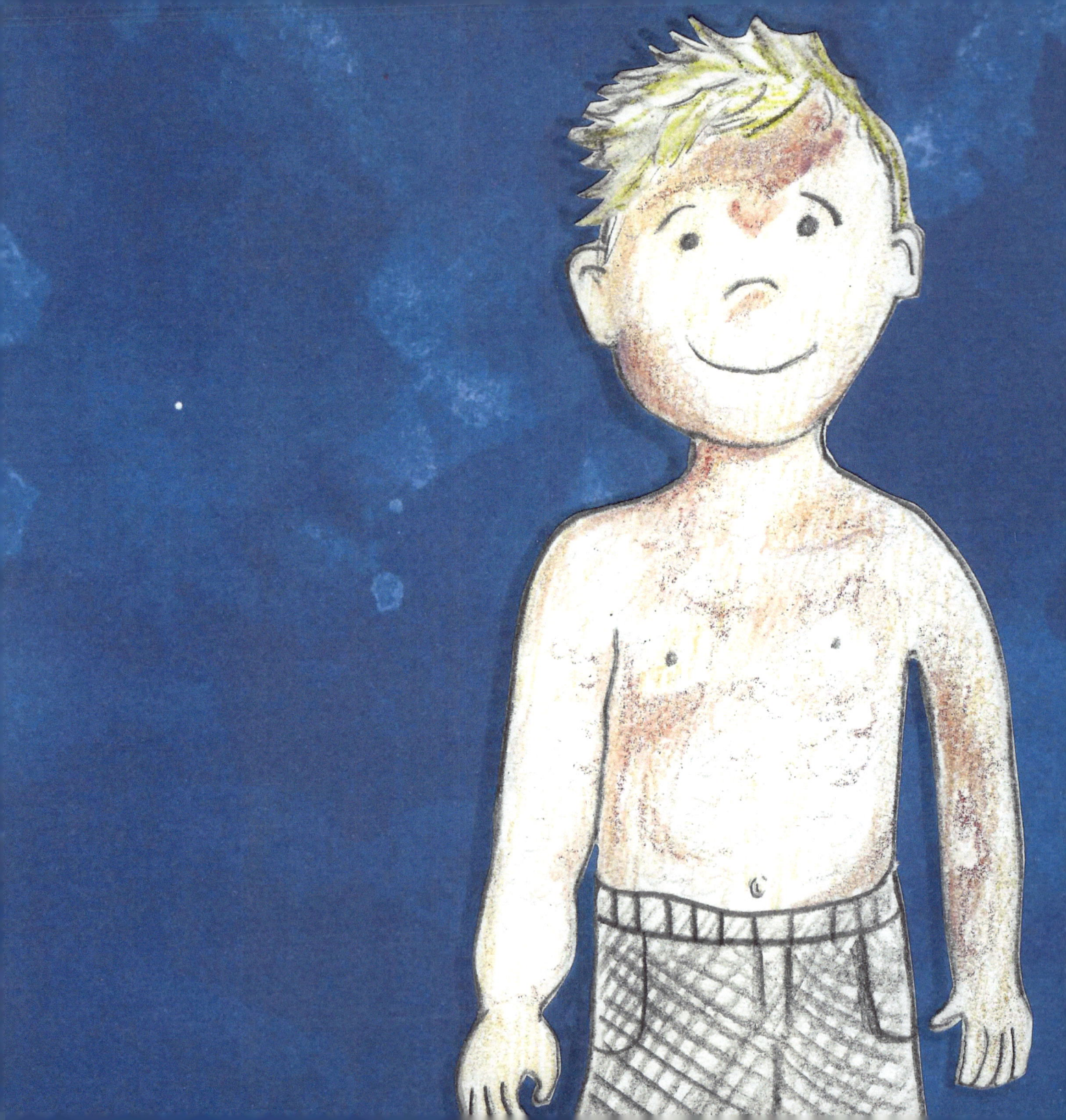

Some of the CHANGED cells show up on
your skin, you can see them-
like a birthmark.

These are called
CAPILLARY MALFORMATIONS.
(you CAN see your capillaries!)

Capillaries are VERY TINY blood vessels in your
skin. In REGULAR cells on your skin
you CAN NOT see your capillaries.

Some of the **CHANGED** cells
you can NOT see
at all.

(UNLESS YOU HAVE X-RAY VISION!!)

Because they are on the INSIDE of your body.

This is why you have to go to the doctor
a lot

The doctor uses different machines and things
to look at your insides and make sure they are
all
working okay.

If the doctor ever sees something that is not working very good, the doctor can do surgery -and fix it- and make it all better.

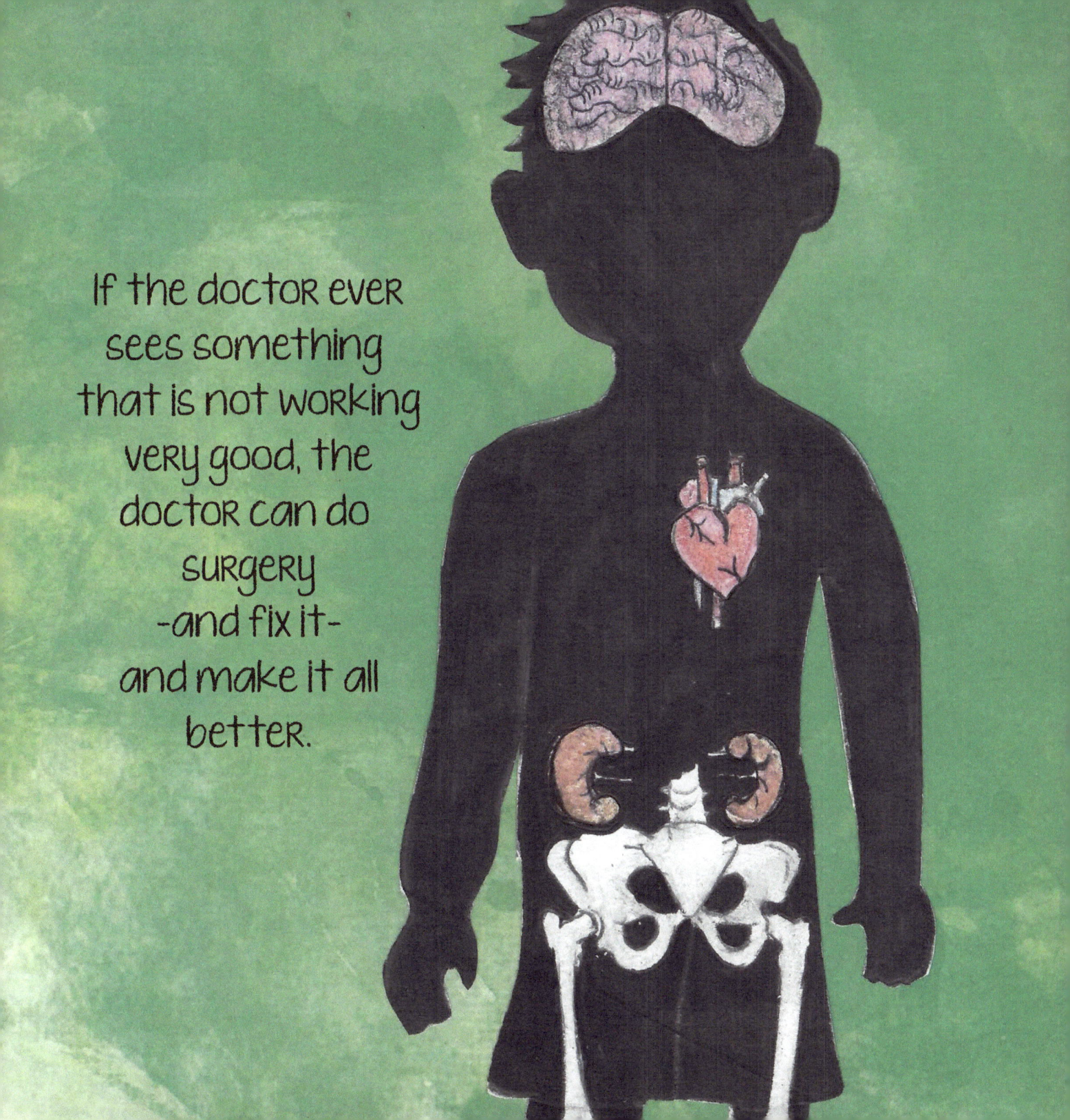

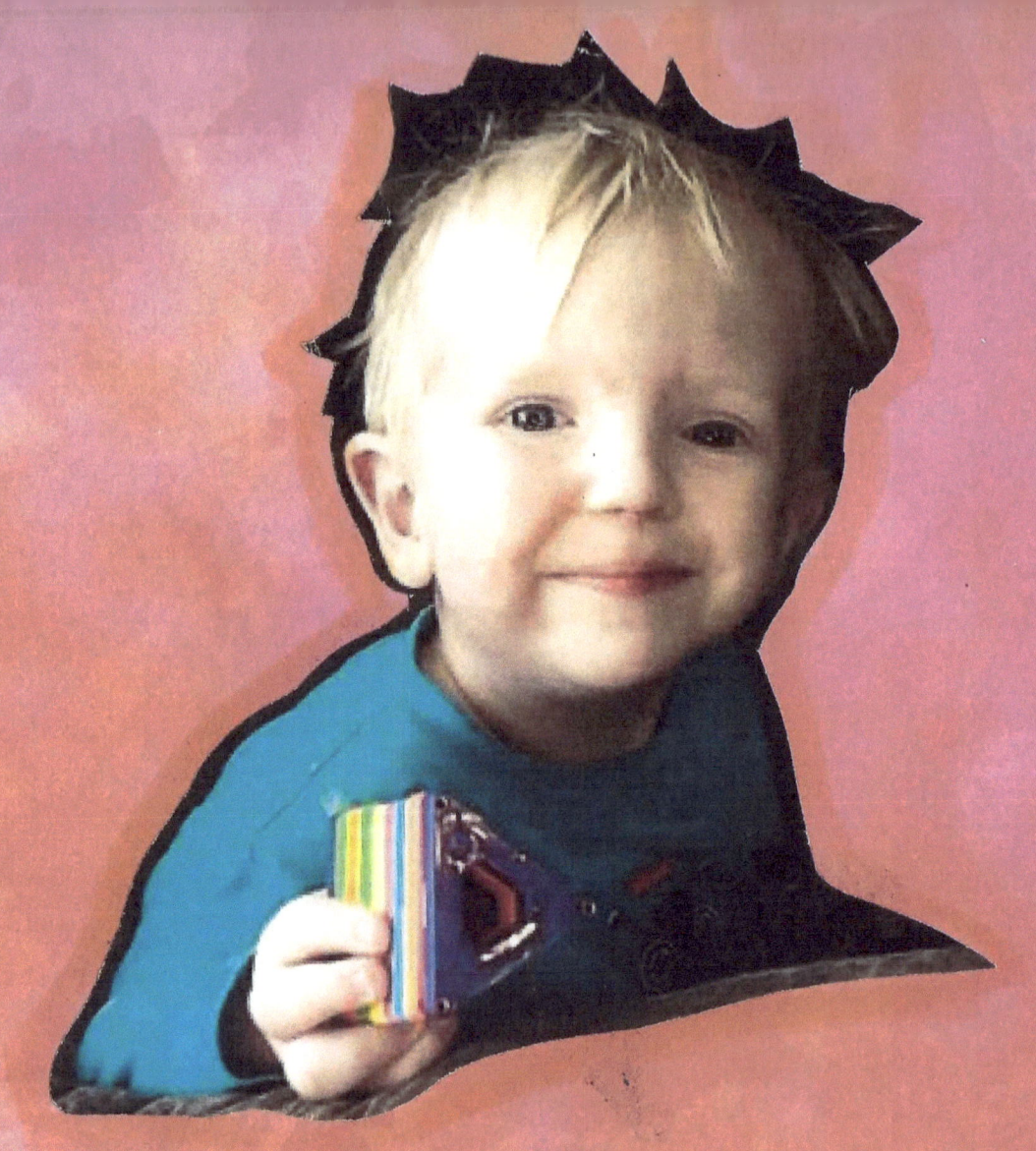

I know this all kinda sounds scary,
but don't be afraid.

This just means that
inside your body you have TWO kinds of cells
that make you special.

Every single person
in the whole wide world
has their very own
DNA.

And everyone's DNA is completely different.

Which means,
Every single person
in the whole wide world
is
DIFFERENt.

God makes each of us
special
AND
unique
AND
different
AND
perfect.

We are made perfect in HIS eyes.

You. Are. Perfect.

PSALM 139:14

I WILL PRAISE YOU FOR I AM FEARFULLY AND WONDERFULLY MADE.

In the original Hebrew text, the word 'wonderfully' means: unique, set apart, uniquely marvelous. WOW! No wonder the psalmist bursts out with exuberant praise in Psalm 139:14. He realized the great love and concern that went into his unique and very individual creation. According to this Scripture, you.. me... WE... truly are a Master Piece!

The next time you have the temptation to ask the Lord, "Don't you care what is happening to me?" Remember this verse, because the truth is that He cares and loves you with an acute intensity that cannot ever be measured.